Hydrogen Pe

Miracle Healers From The Kitchen

By
Sharon Daniels

Legal Disclaimers and Notices

Copyright © 2013 Sharon Daniels & Internet Niche Publishers- All rights reserved.

This book contains material protected under International and Federal Copyright laws and treaties. Any unauthorized reprint or use of this material is prohibited. Violators will be prosecuted to the fullest extent of the law.

The author, publishers and distributors of this product assume no responsibility for the use or misuse of this product, or for any physical or mental injury, damage and/or financial loss sustained to persons or property as a result of using this system.

The content of this book is for informational purpose only and use thereof is solely at your own risk. Readers should always consult with a physician before taking any actions of any kind relating to their health. The author, nor the publisher will in no way be held responsible for any reader who fails to do so. Any action taken based on these contents is at the sole discretion and liability of the reader.

Other Books by Sharon Daniels

If you enjoyed this book, you might also like other books from the Miracle Healers From The Kitchen Series

<u>Cayenne Pepper Cures</u>
<u>Coconut Oil Cures</u>
<u>Apple Cider Vinegar Cures</u>

Table of Contents

What is Hydrogen Peroxide? 7
Hydrogen Peroxide's Discovery 9
How is Hydrogen Peroxide Made? 10
Hydrogen Peroxide in Nature 11
    Other Forms of Naturally Occurring Hydrogen Peroxide 11
Peroxide in Medical History 14
    Hydrogen Peroxide and Nose and Throat Conditions 14
    Treatment for Cough and Fever 14
    Treatment of Influenzal Pneumonia 15
    Hydrogen Peroxide and Arterial Plaque Removal 16
    Treatment of Various Heart Conditions 16
    Dr. Otto Warburg's Theory 18
Dr. Farr's Peroxide Experiments 20
    Allergy and Autoimmune System Experiment 21
    Case Study: Treatment for Temporal Arthritis 22
    Case Study: Treatment for Shingles 22
    Case Study: Chronic Obstructive Pulmonary Disease 23
    Case Study: Chronic Yeast Infections 24
    Case Study: Influenza 25
    Case Study: Arteriosclerosis, Stroke and Heart Disease 25
    How Were Farr's Treatments Administered and Measured? 26
    Farr's Explanation: Why H2O2 Treatment Works 27
Bill Munro's H2O2 Inhalation Therapy 28
What Diseases Can Hydrogen Peroxide Treat? 31
    Metabolism 32
    Breathing and Respiratory Problems and Diseases 32
    Heart Problems and Diseases 33
    A brief note on arteriosclerosis (clogged arteries) 34
    Head and Brain Conditions and Diseases 35

Immune Response	36
Bacterial Illnesses	37
Viral Illnesses	38
Pain Related Illnesses and Conditions	40
Blood and Skin Conditions and Diseases	41
H2O2 Therapy and Cancer	43
Recent Studies Published on H2O2 Therapy and Cancer	43
Differences between Food Grade Hydrogen Peroxide and Topical Hydrogen Peroxide	45
Food Grade Hydrogen Peroxide (FGHP)	45
Household Hydrogen Peroxide	46
Medical Application of Hydrogen Peroxide	47
Common Uses for 3 Percent (Store Bought) Hydrogen Peroxide	47
Different Grades of Hydrogen Peroxide and Their Uses	53
Safe Administration of Hydrogen Peroxide Therapy	55
Inhalation Method	55
Transdermal Application	55
Vaporizer Method	55
Topical Application	56
Douche	56
Proper Dilution for Food Grade Hydrogen Therapy	57
Duration of H2O2 Therapy	58
Storage and Safety Tips	59
First Aid and Emergency Procedures	61
Conclusion	63
Online Sources	64
Book Sources	67
Journal Sources	67

What is Hydrogen Peroxide?

Hydrogen peroxide is a colorless, transparent, bitter-tasting liquid at room temperature. It also occurs naturally in gas form, in the air we breathe. Impure hydrogen peroxide is an unstable compound, and readily breaks down into oxygen and water depending on the temperature of its surroundings.

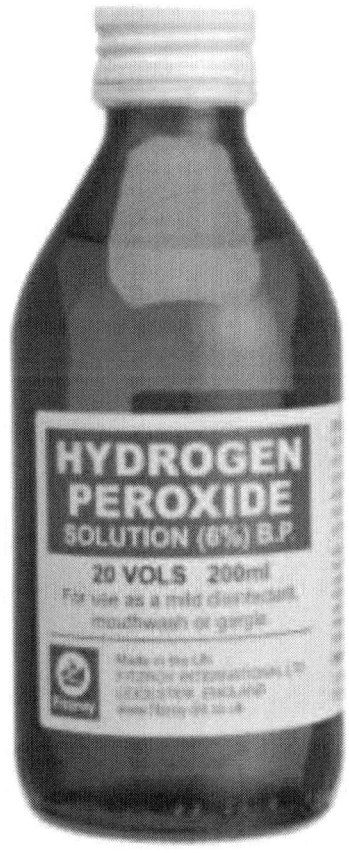

According to the book "Chemical Compounds," written by Schlager and Weisblatt, **pure hydrogen peroxide, unlike regular hydrogen peroxide, is stable**. It only takes a minuscule amount of contamination from copper or iron to change its chemical structure, causing it to rapidly decompose into water and oxygen.

In order to prevent the decomposition of hydrogen peroxide, **elements such as sodium stannate or acetanilide are added.** These compounds act as inhibitors, and are added to various types of hydrogen peroxide solutions and pure forms of hydrogen peroxide.

Hydrogen peroxide on its own is not flammable; however, it can combust when exposed to organic material.

Most households in America contain hydrogen peroxide. These lower concentrations range from 3 to 9 percent, and **many people use them as all-natural bleaches for clothes and hair. In the manufacturing industry, higher concentrations of hydrogen peroxide are used to bleach textiles and paper.** It is also used in the production of organic chemicals, as well as foam and rubber. It is even one of the main components used in rocket fuels.

Hydrogen Peroxide's Discovery

Louis Jacque Thenard was a dedicated chemist and researcher. He discovered hydrogen peroxide in 1818. A hydrogen peroxide molecule consists of both oxygen and hydrogen atoms, which are abundant on Earth.

Low concentrations of hydrogen peroxide can be found within the environment, while gaseous forms are created by photochemical reactions in Earth's atmosphere. Low concentrations of hydrogen peroxide are also found in water.

Hydrogen peroxide was first used commercially during the 1800s; primarily as a bleaching agent for hats. In today's day and age, industrial processes make over 1 billion pounds of hydrogen peroxide each year for many different uses. It is used in everything from teeth whitening products to rocket fuel.

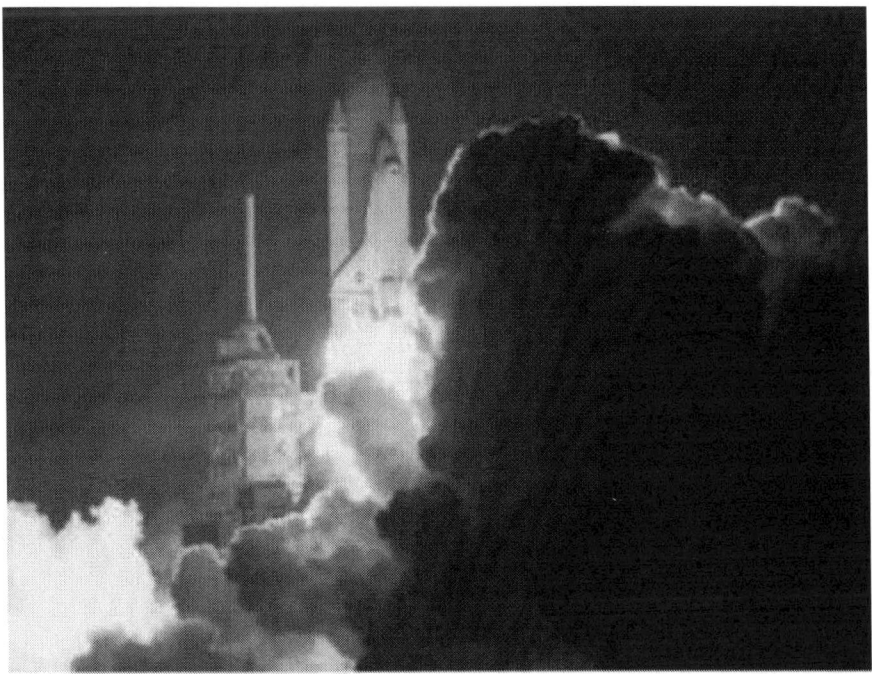

How is Hydrogen Peroxide Made?

Hydrogen peroxide is two-parts hydrogen and two-parts oxygen. Its chemical formula is **H2O2**. Because of its instability, **hydrogen peroxide switches from liquid to gas, depending on the temperature of its environment.** The freezing temperature of hydrogen peroxide is just lightly below water's freezing point. The decomposition of hydrogen peroxide is an extremely slow process, which can take place under normal conditions and can be slowed by refrigerating the compound.

Industrial quantities of hydrogen peroxide are created from a sequence of reactions that occur with relative compounds from the alkyl anthrahydroquinones family. Anthrahydroquinones are compounds made up of three rings, which can convert and revert between two and/or more identical structures (Schlager & Weisblatt, 364). Hydrogen peroxide is created as a byproduct that is released when anthrahydroquinones are converting or reverting into different structures. Since anthrahydroquinones are always being restored during the creation of hydrogen peroxide, it is a very efficient process.

Another method of making hydrogen peroxide is when electrolysis of sulfuric acid occurs, which produces a related compound known as proxy-sulfuric acid. Once this compound makes contact with water, it forms hydrogen peroxide.

Hydrogen peroxide can also be created by heating isopropyl alcohol at high temperatures and under high pressure (Schlager & Weisblatt, 364).

Hydrogen Peroxide in Nature

Gaseous hydrogen peroxide is a natural component of photochemical reactions occurring in the lower atmosphere of the earth. It occurs in both unpolluted and polluted atmospheres. Scientists have also recently discovered that Mars' atmosphere contains hydrogen peroxide molecules.

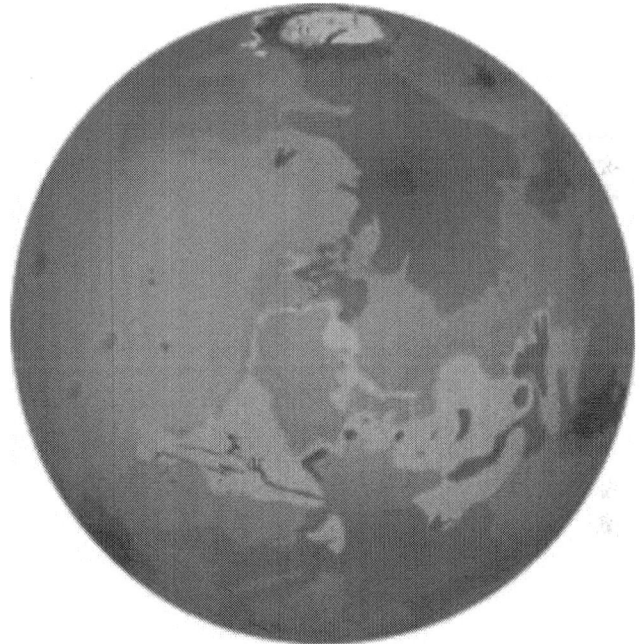

Atmospheric hydrogen peroxide is thought to be created within the remote troposphere via photochemical reactions.

Other Forms of Naturally Occurring Hydrogen Peroxide

Air

- Hydrogen peroxide can be removed from the atmosphere through a process called photolysis, which is the splitting of a chemical compound through light energy or protons.

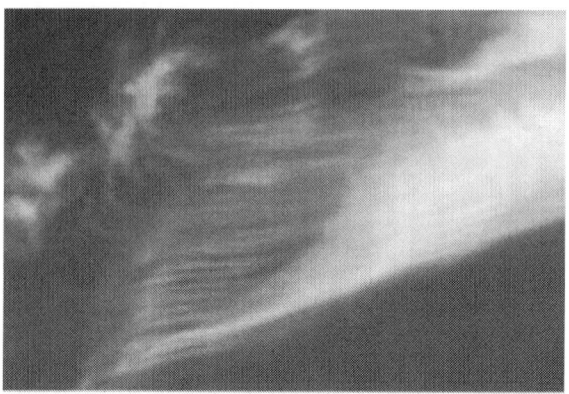

Water

- Surface water concentrations of hydrogen peroxide increase with exposure to sunlight and with contact of dissolved organic matter.

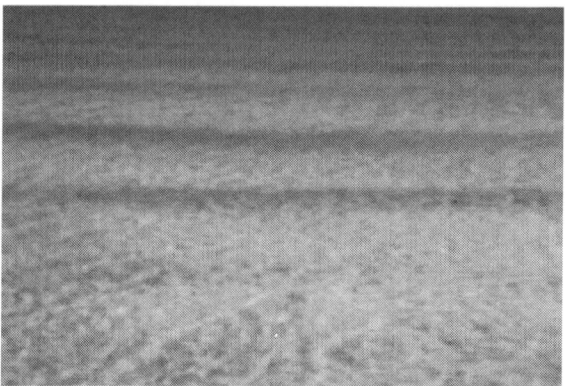

Plant Tissue

- Endogenous hydrogen peroxide - meaning that it arises from causes within an organism - exists inside of plant tissues to varying degrees. Plants that have measurable levels of hydrogen peroxide are green tomatoes, potato tubers, castor beans in water and red tomatoes.

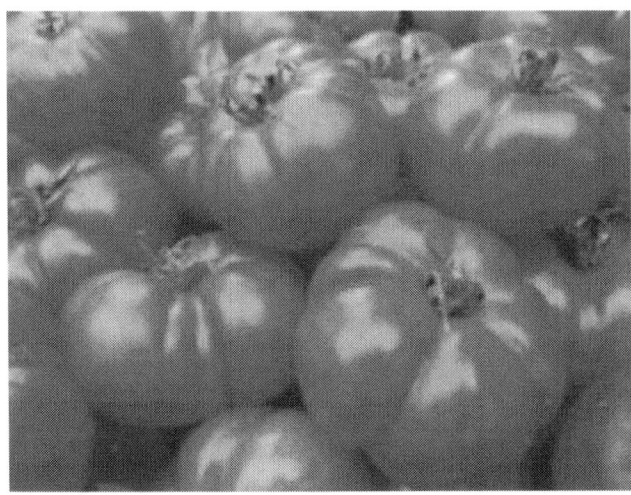

Peroxide in Medical History

Dr. I.N. Love, a physician at the St. Louis City Hospital, performed one of the first documented studies on hydrogen peroxide for medicinal purposes. This study was published in the March 3, 1888 issue of the *Journal of the American Medical Association,* and was titled, "Peroxide of Hydrogen as a Remedial Agent."

The article was influenced by a discussion Love had given at the St. Louis Medical Society one month prior. This discussion highlighted the success of hydrogen peroxide treatment in patients suffering from various diseases. The diseases and illnesses he was able to treat successfully with hydrogen peroxide therapy were whooping cough, hay fever, asthma, tonsillitis, scarlet fever, nasal catarrh, head catarrh, coryza, and diphtheria.

Hydrogen Peroxide and Nose and Throat Conditions

That same year, at the Annual Meeting of the Medical Society of Georgia, Dr. P.R. Cortelyou elaborated upon his scientific findings of using hydrogen peroxide as a way to treat various conditions of the nose and throat.

He diluted a hydrogen peroxide solution with water, and converted it into a fine mist that helped to effectively treat coughs, rhinitis, sore throats, pharyngitis, diphtheria and tonsillitis.

Treatment for Cough and Fever

Dr. Cortelyou also used hydrogen peroxide in conjunction with a variety of other medicines popular during this period. He used a blend of iodine, glycerin, potash and "muriate of cocaine" to help a patient suffering from an acute cough and fever. After four weeks of this treatment, the patient reported feeling significantly better, and the treatment was needed only two times per week thereafter. Dr. Cortelyou also reported that the patient continued feeling good throughout the winter season.

Treatment of Influenzal Pneumonia

British physician T.H. Oliver performed the first documented study of intravenous hydrogen peroxide in 1920. He developed the study following his experiences in India the previous year, where he had treated 25 seriously ill patients with influenzal pneumonia by injecting hydrogen peroxide into their veins.

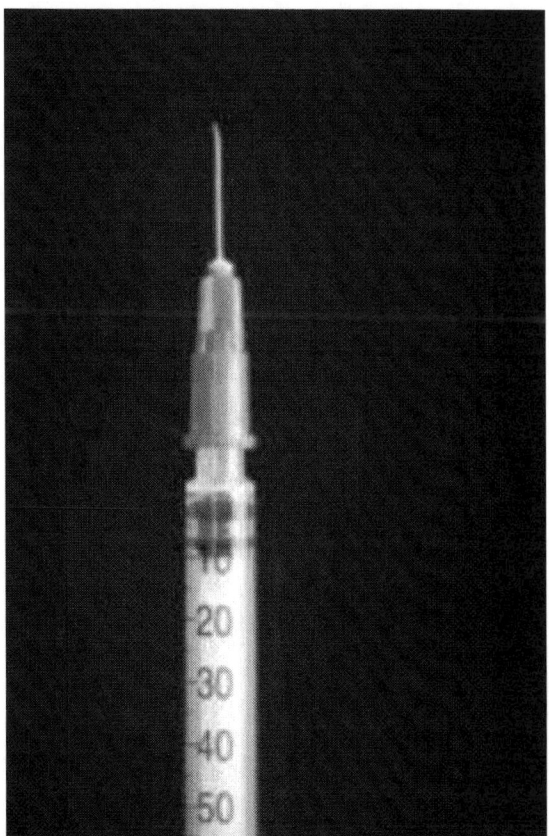

Unfortunately, the normal death rate for influenzal pneumonia was high-- more than 80 percent. What was astonishing was that the death rate of Oliver's patients was significantly lower; only 48% of his patients died.

While the intravenous administration of hydrogen peroxide can be quite dangerous and poses a high risk of stroke in some patients, none of his patients experienced this or any other health problems or complications as a result of this procedure.

Hydrogen Peroxide and Arterial Plaque Removal

Researchers at Baylor University in the 1960's conducted numerous studies on the effects of intravenous hydrogen peroxide on blocked arterial passageways. They discovered that not only was hydrogen peroxide successful at removing plaque buildup in the arteries, but the results were also long-lasting.

While these findings offered an alternative treatment for individuals suffering with this condition; for unknown reasons, they were largely ignored by medical professionals.

Treatment of Various Heart Conditions

In the early 1960's, Baylor University conducted many studies on the medicinal uses of hydrogen peroxide. One of the most important findings made by researchers at this facility was that hydrogen peroxide had a positive effect on the heart muscle. The researchers believed this could benefit patients suffering from cardiovascular problems, such as heart attacks. Myocardial ischemia is a heart condition that occurs when the heart muscle does not receive enough oxygen. Hydrogen peroxide treatment easily relieved this illness.

Dr. H.C. Urschel Jr. wrote in the journal Circulation and reported that ventricular fibrillation, which causes rapid paced incomplete heart contractions of the hollow part of the heart and can be life-threatening, was completely alleviated when patients were given an intravenous solution of hydrogen peroxide.

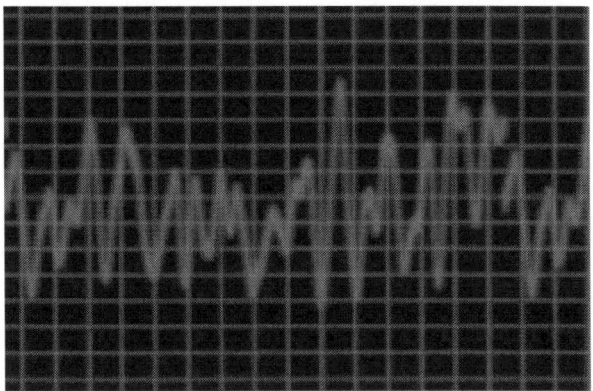

Dr. Otto Warburg's Theory

The belief that hydrogen peroxide could be an effective treatment for cancer was based on a discovery made by Dr. Otto Warburg, a director at the Max Planck Institute for Cell Physiology in Berlin. In 1944, Warburg was once again granted a Nobel Prize for being able to identify enzymes responsible for transferring hydrogen in a wide array of metabolic processes.
However, this wasn't the first time Dr. Warburg was awarded the Nobel Prize. In 1931, Warburg was given the Nobel Prize for his discovery of enzymes that transfer oxygen, a vital process in cellular respiration.

Dr. Warburg's hypothesis for why diseases like cancer develop suggests that cell dysfunction and the inability to process oxygen at the cellular level could be to blame. He believed that metabolic processes of cancerous cells are damaged, and therefore they cannot produce the respiratory functioning needed for extra energy. Warburg also discovered that cancerous cells cannot utilize oxygen to process sugars. Because of this dysfunction, they produce increased amounts of lactic acid and very little energy.

Damaged cells not only contribute to poor functioning of the immune system, but they also create an acidic environment, causing potential damage to DNA and mitochondria, which may lead to cancer and other serious health problems.

In order to better understand what causes diseases like cancer, let's take an in depth look at the molecules responsible for creating damage to cells within the body.

Free Radicals

Dr. Denham Harman was responsible for the free-radical theory on aging, which emerged in the 1950's. The best way to describe free radicals is that they are molecules that have an attached chemically active oxygen atom. Free radicals can cause damage to cells and are responsible for the aging process and various forms of cancer.

At first glance, it appeared as though an abundance of oxygen within the body was detrimental to overall health, and that antioxidants were beneficial to health, especially in regards to protecting the body against accelerated aging.

However, it now appears that not all of the reactions that occur due to free radicals are entirely bad. For example, oxygen aids cleansing enzymes to remove toxins within the body. The immune system also utilizes oxygen to attack foreign substances like bacteria. Hydrogen peroxide also activates natural killer cells that help obliterate cancerous cells that spread throughout the body.

Oxygen and Cancer

Otto Warburg was the first scientist to discover the difference between the metabolic process of cancerous cells and healthy cells. Healthy cells are aerobic, meaning they utilize oxygen in most of their reactions. Cancer cells, on the other hand, are anaerobic, meaning they do not utilize oxygen in their chemical reactions, and therefore, thrive in an oxygen-deprived environment.

The primary energy source for healthy and unhealthy cells is glucose. Cancerous cell have been known to have a huge appetite for glucose when compared to normal cellular metabolism.

How it Works

Intravenous hydrogen peroxide is believed to be successful for treating cancer because it releases pure oxygen in the body. By providing the cells and tissues with high-levels of oxygen, $H2O2$ helps to promote a healthy oxygen-enriched environment, which stimulates the detoxification of oxidative enzymes.

Dr. Farr's Peroxide Experiments

According to the article, "Hydrogen Peroxide: Medical Miracle," written by Dr. William Campbell Douglass, in the 1980's and 1990's, Dr. Charles Farr performed numerous studies on hydrogen peroxide, which were published in a variety of journals. Farr's main goal was to disprove the popular belief that oxygen administered intravenously is completely dissipated in the lungs. Many people believed that the oxygen released by hydrogen peroxide would be expelled into the air. While there is reason to believe that some oxygen would be lost, there is no evidence to support this theory.

In one of Farr's experiments, H2O2 was administered to subjects intravenously in the arm. With this experiment, Farr discovered that patients' metabolic rate had increased significantly, dilation of small arteries had occurred, and oxygen from the hydrogen peroxide infusions remained within the body and circulatory system. As he had suspected, it was not expelled into the air.

Other benefits that that Farr's patients experienced from this experiment included increased mental alertness, better vision, and a feeling of relaxation. Farr and his researchers also reported that many patients suffering from infections, influenza and allergies noticed a significant improvement in the symptoms of these ailments.

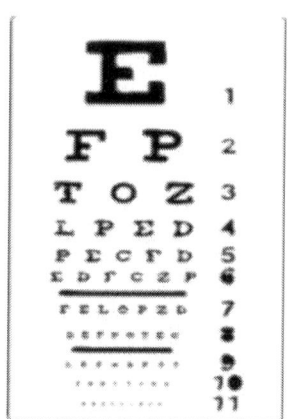

Furthermore, Dr. Farr made another amazing discovery after rendering patients with additional intravenous treatments of hydrogen peroxide. He noted that these patients noticed a vast improvement in their food and pollen related allergies. Dr. Farr also noted that patients with breathing problems such as allergic bronchitis, chronic sinusitis and asthma experienced an improvement in these conditions.

With these findings, Dr. Farr decided to investigate the effects of intravenous hydrogen peroxide treatment on **immune globin fractions and serum anti-body titres. Immune globin fractions** are a preparation of gamma globulins from a large pool of donors used to immunize hepatitis A, and measles; it is also used to treat immune-deficient patients. **Serum anti-body titres** is a laboratory test that measures the level of antibodies in the blood.

Allergy and Autoimmune System Experiment

To conduct this experiment, Farr randomly selected participants from his clinical population. All of the subjects selected either had autoimmune diseases or allergy symptoms. Certain immune globulins were measured prior to and after the intravenous hydrogen peroxide was administered. The results showed a clinical improvement, which corresponded to the reduction of immune globulins.

In the next study, Farr experimented with the Epstein-Barr virus and Candida antibody titres. These were measured before and after the hydrogen peroxide treatments were administered intravenously. In this study, the patients received 20 weekly treatments, which were administered for different durations. The first round of treatments lasted 10 weeks and patients were given one treatment each week; then the subjects received no treatments for an entire month. Once the month of no treatment had passed, subjects were then given another 10-week treatment series. To test the validity of the study, antibody titres were measured four different times; once in the beginning, another after the 20th treatment was rendered, and then again at 90 days and 180 days.

The results showed that all patients experienced a reduction in antibody titres. The patients who previously suffered from Epstein-Barr virus (EBV) reported a significant improvement in their energy and endurance levels and even noticed a reduction in fatigue. The Candida patients also experienced a significant reduction in their Candida antibody titres from the hydrogen peroxide treatment.

Case Study: Treatment for Temporal Arthritis

You may or may not have heard of temporal arthritis, which is diagnosed by severe pain and extreme tenderness of the main superficial artery located near the temple. It's a serious health condition that can eventually lead to blindness if it is not diagnosed and treated promptly.

In 1960, Dr. Farr helped treat an elderly woman suffering from temporal arthritis. While she suffered for many years with this disease, she did not lose her sight, and she found relief through cortisone treatments. However, after several years of cortisone treatments, she developed inflammation of her pancreas, ulcers and colitis.

The elderly woman then switched to a different kind of treatment, known as chelation therapy, which worked for several years but suddenly ceased to be effective. She was once again stricken with painful headaches, and her temporal arthritis eventually returned. Knowing that she couldn't go back to her original form of treatment without sacrificing her health even further, she reached out to Dr. Farr.

Dr. Farr recommended that she undergo a hydrogen peroxide treatment. He went on to explain that $H2O2$ treatment had been shown to be an effective treatment for many inflammatory diseases such as asthma and pneumonia. Since temporal arthritis is the inflammation of the temporal artery, he believed that the hydrogen peroxide therapy would alleviate her symptoms.

Within a few hours of an intravenous $H2O2$ drip, she experienced considerable relief. After a second treatment a week later, she reported feeling completely better.

Case Study: Treatment for Shingles

Shingles occurs when there is an inflammation of the nerve endings, which is caused by the same virus as chicken pox - varicella. Unsightly, painful, puss-filled blisters appear near the skin along the nerve of the spine. While there are many treatments for this condition, none of them have been able to get rid of the virus. What makes shingles painful to live with, is that it can last for an extended period of time – for years in extreme cases - and wreak havoc on the individuals who suffer from it.

Dr. Farr was successful in treating an elderly man with severe shingles on his upper body. After three days of an infused hydrogen peroxide treatment, the patient was noticeably better and one week later he was free from pain. The blisters also started to dry up. Dr. Farr stated that many therapeutic modalities had been used to treat shingles; however, each one had varying success rates. By using the hydrogen peroxide treatment, the patient experienced results that were up to three-times faster than any other existing treatment method.

Case Study: Chronic Obstructive Pulmonary Disease

Chronic Obstructive Pulmonary Disease (COPD) causes the bronchial tubes to close and makes breathing a constant chore for those stricken with this condition. Another consequence of COPD is the accumulation of mucous and pus that blocks the respiratory passages, which can result in death. Scarring can potentially occur due to the constant, acute inflammation and spasms of the bronchial passages.

A patient suffering from COPD was given intravenous hydrogen peroxide therapy. After a few minutes of receiving the treatment, the patient started coughing profusely and began spitting up yellow mucous. What Dr. Farr noticed was that the coughing and mucous production was influenced by the hydrogen peroxide therapy and he could control the patient's coughing by either halting or administering the administration of H_2O_2.

Dr. Farr defined this term as "effervescent debridement." Oxygen seeps into air pockets beneath the layer of mucous and causes it to loosen and bubble. The patient then coughs, and this provides the momentum needed to expel the mucous from the body.

What's even more amazing is that this same patient suffered from chronic diarrhea for more than two years; not only did this subside, but she also no longer experienced migratory arthritis or muscle pain, unrelated conditions which has also affected her.

Case Study: Chronic Yeast Infections

Candidiasis is a yeast infection that stems from an overgrowth of fungus within the body.
There are over 20 different species of this type of fungi. They can live on any surface of the body and can multiply at an incredibly fast rate, especially given the right (warm, moist) conditions. When this occurs, an infection is likely to set in.

Common forms of these infections are vaginal yeast infections, diaper rash, thrush and infections of the nail bed.

Some people who have taken antibiotics to kill infections in other areas of the body may be prone to developing recurring yeast infections. This happens because antibiotics kill bacteria indiscriminately, including the species which protect us from certain ailments.

This is what happened to one of Dr. Farr's patients, a middle-aged woman who suffered from yeast syndrome.

One of Dr. Farr's patients, a middle-aged woman, began suffering from yeast syndrome after she received prolonged treatment with antibiotics, which were used to help fight chronic lung infections she had been experiencing. Some of her symptoms included chronic yeast infections, diarrhea, headaches, acne, arthritis and concentration problems.

She had tried just about every form of therapy and treatment to help with these infections. While the treatments did offer temporary relief, the infections continued to return, time and time again. Eventually she became incapacitated and needed round-the-clock-care, provided by her mother.

What was really quite impressive was that after Dr. Farr had given her two intravenous hydrogen peroxide treatments, she reported feeling better.

She also stated that she noticed a vast improvement in her alertness and an improvement in her ability to concentrate.

The woman noticed a vast improvement in her acne and even noticed an increased level in her strength. After she received eight hydrogen peroxide treatments, she no longer experienced any symptoms.

A follow-up was conducted two months later, and the patient showed no visible signs of Candidiasis. Her allergy to yeast had also significantly improved, a fact which was confirmed by a skin test.

Case Study: Influenza

One of the most popular documented uses of hydrogen peroxide for medicinal purposes is to treat influenza and other respiratory infections.

Dr. Farr documented an example of hydrogen peroxide treatment working to treat the flu virus when he gave an elderly man suffering from symptoms of influenza an H2O2 drip treatment. Before the patient received H2O2 therapy, he had a fever of 102 degrees Fahrenheit. A day after he was given the treatment, his temperature had dropped to 101 degrees Fahrenheit. He was then administered another H2O2 treatment. Before the second infusion was finished, his temperature returned to normal and he no longer exhibited symptoms of the flu.

Case Study: Arteriosclerosis, Stroke and Heart Disease

According to the U.S. National Library of Medicine, coronary heart disease, also known as CHD, is the leading cause of death in both American men and women. This disease causes tapering of the tiny blood vessels that supply oxygen and blood to the heart; thus preventing the flow of blood and oxygen to the heart.

A 71-year-old patient, by the name of Mr. J.H. was being treated for heart disease at the clinic in Oklahoma City where Dr. Farr worked. After receiving 11 treatments of chelation therapy the patient started exhibiting symptoms of a stroke. His speech slurred, he had blurry vision and he began drooling from the mouth.

When Dr. Farr examined him, he noticed that the patient was not only confused and showed signs of being disoriented. Farr knew that the patient was at risk of dying.

Instead of referring the patient to a neurologist, who would have had nothing definitive to offer the patient, Dr. Farr took matters into his own hands and immediately administered an intravenous infusion of hydrogen peroxide. Fifteen minutes later, the patient's speech improved and he was no longer confused or disoriented. An hour later, his symptoms had diminished entirely.

How Were Farr's Treatments Administered and Measured?

In his first experiment, Farr utilized three different methods to measure the results he obtained. One of the instruments that Farr used measured oxygen consumption. Patients had to wear a mask over their faces while a computer calculated the amount of oxygen they inhaled and exhaled. The computer then provided results based on the difference between the two. When the patient's weight is known, it is easy to determine the rate that the body is using oxygen. This process is called measuring the metabolic rate of the body. If the metabolic rate rises once the hydrogen peroxide therapy is administered, then Farr's hypothesis is correct, and more oxygen is making its way into the tissues.

In Farr's treatment, less than a few minutes after receiving the infusion, the metabolic rate started to rise. The metabolism rose to 100 percent and stayed there until the infusion was no longer rendered, and the metabolic rate returned to baseline after 30 minutes had elapsed.

Another experiment involved measuring the change of the temperature on the surface of the body, as a result of vasodilatation - the dilation of the tiny blood vessels in the skin.

Farr gauged the effectiveness of the treatment on the patients by measuring their temperature. If body temperature rose during the treatment, then oxygenation was accomplished and vasodilatation had taken place. Therefore, the blood vessels would dilate, circulation would improve and more oxygen would make its way into the tissues. After 10 minutes of receiving the infusion, the temperature of the body surface had risen by one degree, which corresponded with vasodilatation and an increase in oxygen consumption.

All of the measurements taken, including oxygen consumption, temperature, and dilation of blood vessels, were duplicated for a period of 6 consecutive days for all of the patients.

Very few treatments in the world of medicine are able to be repeated and are as easy to determine as Farr's peroxide treatment. What makes the hydrogen peroxide therapy results so groundbreaking is that so few therapies offer this kind of reliability. Medical treatments either work or they don't; there is no mystery involved.

Farr's Explanation: Why H2O2 Treatment Works

While some studies support and confirm the theory that H2O2 administered intravenously would cause hydrogen peroxide to release oxygen, which would then be completely expelled by the lungs, Dr. Farr set out to prove otherwise. If this hypothesis and its supporting studies were the only viable explanation of how the body processes H2O2, he couldn't understand how he could have such success with the H2O2 treatments he was administering to patients.

Dr. Farr's explanation for why the hydrogen peroxide treatments were so successful has to do with the way they were administered and the length of time it took them to begin working. Many of the treatments he performed with hydrogen peroxide were given intravenously or directly into the tissue, but there was a 40 minute delay in the rise of oxygen levels. This supported his theory that H2O2 that is injected into the veins does not immediately breakdown into H2O and O2; therefore, the O2 would not be immediately exhaled out of the lungs.

Bill Munro's H2O2 Inhalation Therapy

Please note that hydrogen peroxide at doses higher than 3 percent if not properly diluted can be dangerous. This method, while promising, has not been tested in medical studies.

PROCEED AT YOUR OWN RISK.

Mr. Bill Munro, from Waterford, MI, states that he has been inhaling 3 percent hydrogen peroxide for over 13 years. A regular everyday consumer like you and me, Mr. Munro was fed up with his inability to breathe clearly and was unable to do the many things he wanted to do around the house, without having to deal with shortness of breath and painful, tight joints.

At 69 years old, Mr. Munro was dealing with several health issues, most of which were consequences of aging. He noticed that he started experiencing acute tightness in his muscles, which made it difficult to sit up, stand, or walk. In fact, he was finding trouble every day just trying to get out of bed.

Mr. Munro knew he had to do something about his daily difficulties, but he didn't know exactly what. Then one day, a friend came to visit, and brought a stack of books with him. One of the books that piqued Mr. Munro's interest was a book on oxygen therapy. While the book covered a vast array of oxygen therapies, the only one that appealed to Mr. Munro was the inhalation method.

Mr. Munro found a nasal spray pump; it was the perfect tool to help him inhale 3 percent hydrogen peroxide. At first, Mr. Munro settled for one pump per inhalation; he administered this treatment about 4 times a day, for about a month. He began to notice that he could breathe freely – he no longer had to force oxygen in or out of his lungs as his breathing was no longer labored.

After he noticed what type of results the hydrogen peroxide had on his breathing, he decided to increase his dose to 2 pumps per inhalation in the morning and at night. He was soon able to sleep the entire night with his mouth closed, and he no longer experienced the chest pains he used to deal with every night.

Unfortunately, during this same time period, Mr. Munro had been diagnosed with melanoma and prostate cancers. After hearing this disturbing news, Mr. Munro felt like it was time to take action against these growths. Since he had experienced such tremendous success with the hydrogen peroxide treatment with his other health ailments, Mr. Munro decided to increase his dose of hydrogen peroxide treatment to help cure his cancers. He was also very careful not to allow anything to come into contact with his melanoma, because he knew that this would keep the flow of oxygen from making its way to the sore and delay the healing processes from the outside.

In order to increase the amount of oxygen on the inside, he increased the number of his inhalations from 7 to 8 times a day. With each inhalation, he would pump the nasal spray dispenser 10 times. He did this for a period of about four months. He has since decreased his pumping to 5 times a day with each inhale, with 7 treatments per day. To his amazement, his most recent PSA blood tests also showed that he was free of prostate cancer.

Mr. Munro believes that in order to see vast results, you need to administer the peroxide treatment at least 5 to 6 times daily. According to this treatment, Mr. Munro states that within 2 to 4 weeks viruses will be destroyed. He also states that while cancer takes about a month to get rid of, you would need to continue the hydrogen peroxide therapy for at least 3 to 4 months. He believes that viruses cannot survive in an environment where oxygen is abundant.

Mr. Munro states that any time he feels muscle spasms coming on from doing too much hard work, he takes out his nasal pump and inhales the peroxide. Within one minute, he notices that the muscle spasms stop.

Now 78 years old, Mr. Munro says that he and his wife have been inhaling hydrogen peroxide together for the past 9 years. He reports that they have not experienced any colds, sore muscles, aches or pains since beginning this therapy. He also went on to add that he doesn't even take any medications or vitamins.

What Diseases Can Hydrogen Peroxide Treat?

Hydrogen peroxide can be used to treat a wide variety of diseases due to its antiseptic properties; it kills bacteria viruses, parasites and fungi. The compound even has the ability to obliterate certain cells that cause tumors.

Hydrogen peroxide is just as – if not more – important than the thyroid in maintaining stable body temperature. This is a result of the molecule's role in intracellular thermogenesis - which is the technical name for cell warming - and is vital to all of life's processes.

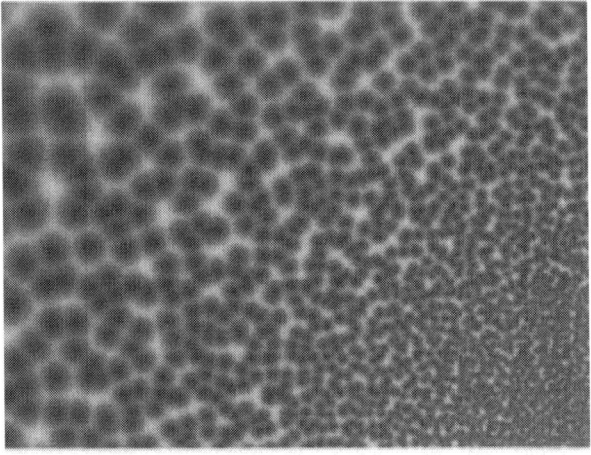

Numerous experiments on the effects of hydrogen peroxide in animals have shown that the organs with the highest concentration of this substance were the lungs, thymus, intestine, kidneys and liver. This suggests that these organs easily absorb hydrogen peroxide.

The following effects of H2O2 have been studied in the medical literature, observed by regular users of H2O2, or are currently being investigated.

Metabolism

- Hydrogen peroxide occurs naturally as part of the metabolic process. It is quickly decomposed by catalase, one of the most efficient enzymes found in healthy cells.

- Gluthathione peroxides are the main components responsible for the decomposition of hydrogen peroxide. They are present in healthy human tissues.

- When hydrogen peroxide and catalase are exposed to one another, the hydrogen peroxide quickly decomposes into water and oxygen.

Breathing and Respiratory Problems and Diseases

Conditions treated:

- Allergies
- Asthma
- Emphysema
- Chronic Obstructive Pulmonary Diseases

Food grade hydrogen peroxide (FGHP) treatment has been shown to be effective for various types of breathing and respiratory problems. This is because it helps to break up mucous and other debris deep within the lungs and air pathways that cause breathing problems. Once the debris is loosened, it makes it easier for the patient to cough up and expel it from the body. This helps clear air passages and improve breathing.

There is reason to believe that hydrogen peroxide treatment can also help people breathe better. This is because once the debris or phlegm from within the lungs is expelled, the air passages are cleared and breathing is improved. Most hydrogen peroxide users report being able to breathe better and some even notice a vast improvement in the clarity of their sinuses.

$H2O2$ treatment helps with other breathing and respiratory problems by stimulating oxygenation in the lungs via improved blood flow. Hydrogen peroxide assists the hemoglobin in red blood cells transmit oxygen to the lungs, which helps remove foreign debris such as dead and damaged tissue from the alveoli.

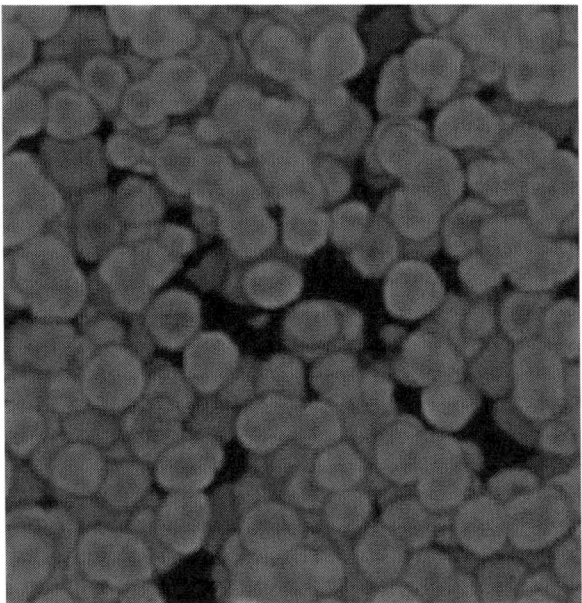

Some of the breathing and respiratory problems that have been treated with FGHP are allergies, asthma, emphysema and Chronic Obstructive Pulmonary Disease.

Intra-nasal hydrogen peroxide treatment is beneficial for a variety of other respiratory illnesses and infections. It may also prove effective in the treatment of other health issues, including chronic sinusitis, halitosis (bad breath) and bronchiectasis.

Just as a side note, it should be mentioned that H2O2, while very effective at ridding the lungs of harmful bacteria, cannot undo damage already done to the lungs.

Heart Problems and Diseases

Conditions treated:

- Heart Stoppage (Cardio Conversion)

- Heart Disease (Cardiovascular Disease)
- Irregular Heartbeat (Cardiac Arrhythmias)
- Peripheral Vascular Disease (poor circulation)

Few treatments work as effectively as FGHP at removing plaque within the arteries, which can lead to high cholesterol and high blood pressure. Removing plaque within the arteries helps to improve cardiovascular health and decrease the risk of heart attacks and strokes.

Some of the heart problems and diseases that FGHP has been shown to improve are heart stoppage, irregular heartbeat and peripheral vascular disease. However, even when hydrogen peroxide is not used as a form of medical treatment, it still helps researchers understand more about particular degenerative diseases.

Recent research published in Clinical Chemistry & Laboratory Medicine, was conducted on reactive oxygenation species (ROS). ROS play a vital role in the pathogenesis of degenerative diseases, including atherosclerosis.

In order to come up with a more reliable way of measuring oxidative stress, researchers began evaluating the characteristics of an automated test which measures hydroperoxides (HPs) and their ability to determine the levels of oxidative stress that occurs in the general population suffering from CAD or coronary heart disease. The results showed that hydroperoxides were higher in people with CAD and increased with the severity of this disease. This study supports previous documented research, and implies that hydrogen peroxide is a more accurate and reliable way of measuring oxidative stress that occurs within the body.

A brief note on arteriosclerosis (clogged arteries)

Chelation therapy is an extremely beneficial treatment for people suffering from problems with peripheral circulation. However, one of the downsides to this form of treatment is that it cannot get rid of the hardened plaque found within larger heart arteries, including the aorta.

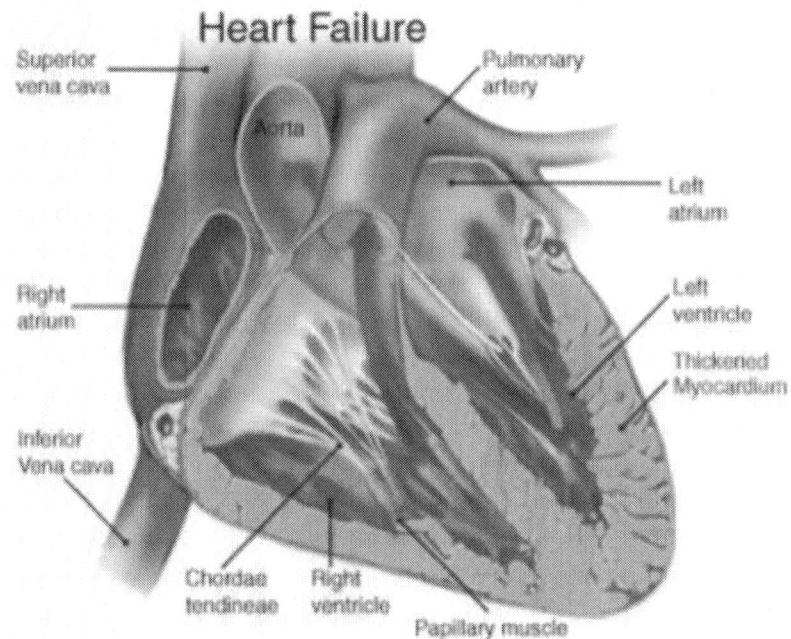

The Medical Center at Baylor University conducted a study on patients who suffered from severe arteriosclerosis. Some patients were given an injection of hydrogen peroxide, while others were not. When these patients died, autopsies were performed to see if there was a difference in the arteries of the patients who received the H2O2 treatment and those who did not. The researchers discovered that the plaque buildup in the blood vessels was absent in the patients who were given the hydrogen peroxide treatment.

Head and Brain Conditions and Diseases

Conditions treated:

- Alzheimer's disease
- Cerebral Vascular disease (stroke and memory loss)
- Cluster headaches
- Migraines
- Multiple Sclerosis
- Parkinson's disease

- Inflammation of the Temporal Artery (Temporal Arthritis)
- Vascular headaches

One of the reasons why FGHP is believed to help reduce migraine headaches and cluster headaches is due to its ability to either increase or decrease the size of blood vessels, depending on environmental controls. Migraine headaches occur as a result of an overproduction of chemicals and the related inflammation of blood vessels near the temples. Hydrogen peroxide is believed to help reduce inflammation that occurs in the temporal artery.

Other head and brain conditions that have been reportedly treated by hydrogen peroxide therapy are Alzheimer's disease, stroke and memory loss, cluster headaches, multiple sclerosis, Parkinson's disease, temporal arthritis and vascular headaches.

Hydrogen peroxide that occurs naturally within the body can also be an indicator of certain diseases and illnesses. It may even help researchers find alternative ways to treat certain age-related diseases like Parkinson's and Alzheimer's disease.

Alzheimer's and Parkinson's diseases are neurodegenerative disorders that cause impairment of motor functions and cognitive impairment, in addition to shortened life spans. In recent times, it has been discovered that these diseases may also overlap. Based on these findings, a new study was conducted where researchers proposed that hydrogen peroxide would be involved in intracellular signalization, which encourages neuron loss in Alzheimer's and Parkinson's diseases.

By conducting this review, researchers have a better understanding of the importance of H2O2-generated by enzymes or metacatalyzed oxidation of dopamine. Therefore, the creation of these chemicals may help researchers find alternative therapeutic strategies for both diseases.

Immune Response

In the Arthritis Trust of America website's article "Supplement to *The Art of Getting Well:* Hydrogen Peroxide Therapy," Drs. Farr and Joseph explain that as we age, our immune system weakens. This allows unhealthy organisms to spread throughout the body and cause a variety of illnesses. By killing these harmful organisms, people can gain temporary relief from microbial warfare and give their immune system the time it needs to recuperate.

Dr. William Campbell Douglass states that hydrogen peroxide helps accomplish two things: it helps to kill foreign bodies, and it helps to prevent the absorption of these foreign germs. Not only does hydrogen peroxide help to kill harmful substances on contact, but it also acts as an important protective barrier by preventing these bacterium from entering the body and causing various illnesses.

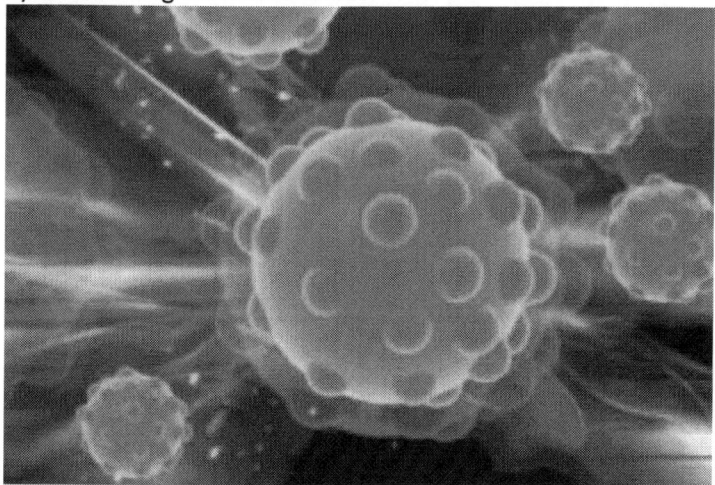

Bacterial Illnesses

Conditions treated:

- Chronic Unresponsive Bacterial Infections
- Parasitic Infections
- Systemic Chronic Candidiasis (yeast infections)

Since food grade hydrogen peroxide or FGHP has antiseptic properties, it kills microbes that are responsible for a variety of illnesses and diseases. Some of the illnesses FGHP has been successful at treating are chronic unresponsive bacterial infections, parasitic infections and yeast infections.

According to the article "Elevated levels of urinary hydrogen peroxide, advanced oxidative protein and malondialdehyde in humans infected with intestinal parasites," oxidative stress is a known indicator of the pathophysiology of numerous fatal illnesses and diseases, including cardiovascular disease, diabetes and cancer. It transpires when free radicals invade the natural antioxidant defenses within the body.

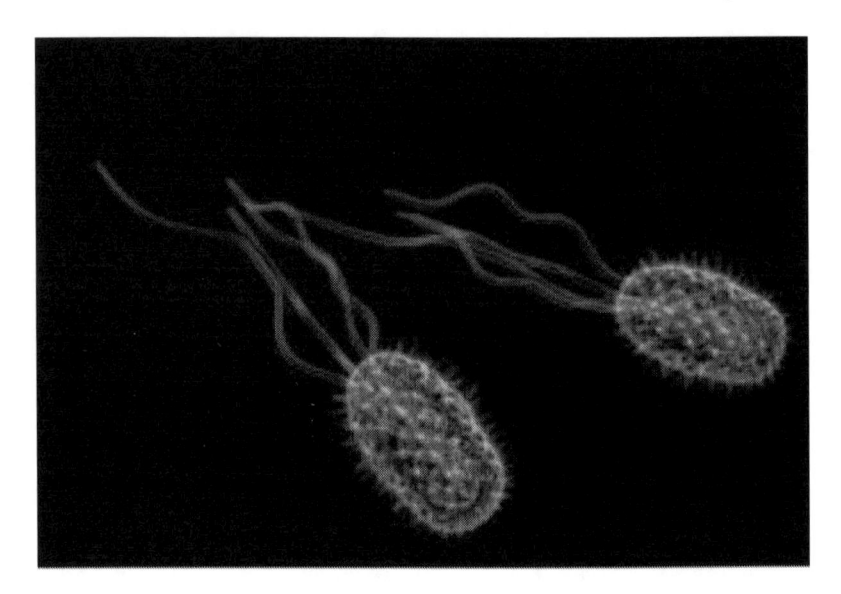

Past research has implied that patients suffering from parasitic infections will also undergo oxidative stress; however, to date there is a lack of sufficient evidence for this theory.

In order to measure whether oxidative stress occurs in patients with intestinal parasites, researchers used three different assays: hydrogen peroxide, lipid per oxidation, and oxidative protein.

The results found that oxidative stress is prominent in subjects who had an infection caused by intestinal parasites. Therefore, hydrogen peroxide helps researchers determine and diagnose whether a patient has intestinal parasites, which can be vital to saving the patient's life and rendering the proper treatment to kill the parasitic infection.

Viral Illnesses

Conditions treated:

- Acute and Chronic Viral Infections
- Fever Blister (Herpes Simplex)
- Influenza (Flu)
- HIV-related illnesses
- Recurrent and Acute Epstein-Barr
- Shingles (Herpes Zoster)

Food grade hydrogen peroxide can be used to kill many different short-term and long-term fatal viruses that wreak havoc on everyday life.

The reason FGHP works at killing viruses is that it supplies the body with the oxygen it needs to fend off viruses, as viruses cannot survive in an oxygen-abundant environment. Some of the viral related illnesses and diseases that have been treated with hydrogen peroxide treatment are herpes simplex, influenza, HIV-related illnesses, acute and recurrent Epstein-Barr virus and shingles.

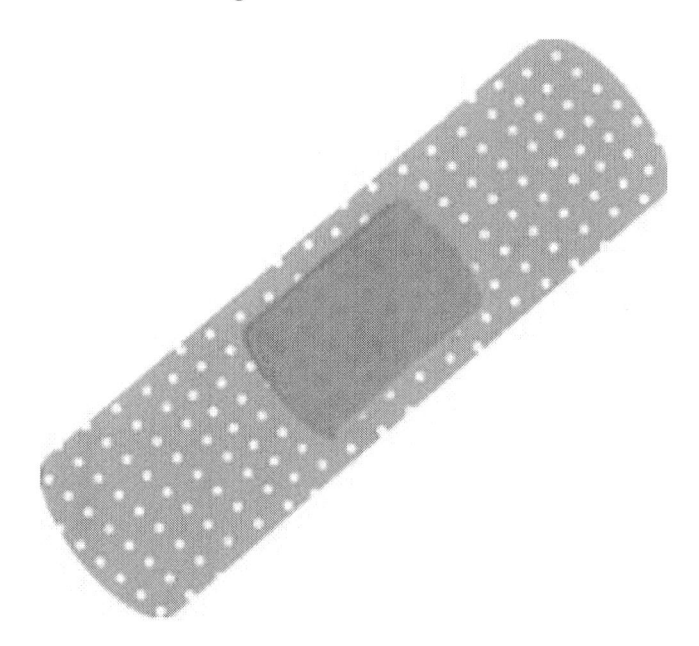

According to the article, "Induction of Interferon-gamma Production by Human Natural Killer Cells Stimulated by Hydrogen Peroxide," published in the Journal of Immunology in 1985, hydrogen peroxide helps to produce gamma interferon, which is a protein that helps promote healing once it is exposed to foreign matter, such as cellular messengers or viruses.

Pain Related Illnesses and Conditions

Conditions treated:

- Chronic Pain Syndrome (from different causes)
- Rheumatoid Arthritis

Food grade hydrogen peroxide therapy has been proven effective in the treatment of a multitude of pain-related illnesses and conditions such as chronic pain syndrome and rheumatoid arthritis. When hydrogen peroxide is injected into the joints it helps to reduce the painful inflammation that commonly occurs with these joint related diseases.

A study published in the Arthritis & Rheumatism in 2011 was conducted on objective neutrophil, which causes the inflammation responsible for rheumatoid arthritis. This study was performed on lab mice and was conducted in order to examine the influence of H2O2 on neutrophilic inflammation.

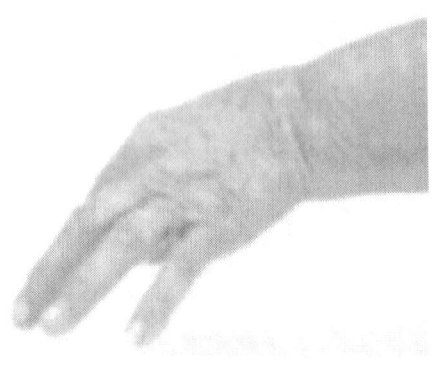

The function of H2O2 was examined by using mice that do not produce ROS and drugs that boost the production or the deprivation of H2O2.

The results showed that H2O2 levels increased during europhile influx, which is imperative for reducing neutrophilic inflammation. Variation of H2O2 production may represent an innovative way of controlling joint inflammation.

Blood and Skin Conditions and Diseases

Conditions treated:

- Diabetes Mellitus II
- Metastatic Carcinoma (Cancer)
- Acne

Diabetes mellitus, cancer and acne are all blood and skin conditions of varying degrees that have been effectively treated with hydrogen peroxide therapy. One reason why hydrogen peroxide is believed to treat acute diseases including cancer is that it provides the body with the amount of oxygen it needs to obliterate cancer cells. Many researchers believe that cancer cells cannot survive or thrive in an oxygen-rich environment.

Another important function that H2O2 therapy provides is that it also helps to increase white blood cell count within the blood. White blood cells are essential for good overall health because they keep the immune system strong and able to fight off various diseases and illnesses.

A study performed by R. Capizzi and F. Landli, which was published in the *British Journal of Dermatology*, August 2004, Volume 151, was conducted to see whether a new treatment cream that utilizes 1 percent hydrogen peroxide and adapalene gel would cause less skin irritation than benzoyl peroxide and adapalene gel in the treatment of acne vulgaris.

The results showed that the 1 percent hydrogen peroxide treatment with adapalene gel caused less skin irritation than the benzoyl peroxide and adapelene gel treatment. The study also showed that the hydrogen peroxide treatment with adapalene was better at reducing inflammation and the number of lesions on the face than the benzoyl peroxide and adapalene gel cream. The study's subjects also experienced more skin dryness and burning sensations with the benzoyl peroxide and adapelene gel treatment than they did with the hydrogen peroxide and adapalene treatment.

In the treatment of diabetes, hydrogen peroxide behaves similarly to insulin, by helping to transport sugar throughout the body.

Glucose oxidase, a once mysterious enzyme, has received a lot of attention due to its role in diabetes. It is used in devices for home blood glucose monitoring, and helps patients monitor the level of glucose in their blood. Serious health consequences can arise if blood glucose levels are too low or too high. These devices help prevent this from happening by using biosensor technology, which measures blood glucose levels in a more accurately than prior methods.

Glucose oxidase causes the conversion process of glucose into glucolactone, which also converts oxygen into hydrogen peroxide. This process is called an oxidation-reduction because molecules experience either a loss or gain of electrons.

The first enzyme used in blood glucose meters was glucose oxidase. In the May 2006 issue of Research Collaboratory for Structural Bioinformatics, David S. Goodsell explains how these devices measure the glucose oxidase reaction. He states that while glucose is difficult to measure, hydrogen peroxide is not. Blood glucose monitors are equipped with an electrode that senses when hydrogen peroxide is formed in the reaction. Therefore, the more peroxide that remains, the more glucose there is within the blood.

There are two types of molecules involved in this process. One is the donor molecule, which is oxidated. The other is the receptor molecule, which is reduced. During the glucose oxidase reaction, the only electron receptor remaining is oxygen, which is then reduced to hydrogen peroxide.

Monitors are essential for diabetics, providing them with more control over their diabetes, since they are able to monitor their blood sugar levels closely. By frequently checking blood sugar levels, diabetics can avoid the long-term complications such as blindness and diabetic ulcers, which can occur as a consequence of poor management of the disease.

H2O2 Therapy and Cancer

As we have seen, hydrogen peroxide plays a crucial role in the human body. It is essential for the proper functioning of cells, and has been used to cure and treat a variety of diseases and health conditions of varying severity.

In the Beginning

As far back as the early 19th century, doctors used H2O2 therapy to treat bacterial infections, including syphilis, which were infections resistant to other forms of treatment. In the beginning of the 20th century, medical doctors used H2O2 therapy to treat a wide array of diseases such as asthma, whooping cough, ulcers, tuberculosis and typhoid fever.

However, for reasons that are unclear today, the success of H2O2 treatment was ignored by many medical professionals and instead high-priced pharmaceuticals were prescribed to patients to treat these same diseases.

In addition to its ability to increase available oxygen and therefore improve cell function in the body, one reason hydrogen peroxide therapy works for treating acute diseases is its strong sterilizing power. H2O2 makes it virtually impossible for diseases and infections to survive. This sterilizing power results from the extra atom of oxygen in the hydrogen peroxide molecule.

Recent Studies Published on H2O2 Therapy and Cancer

Study #1

Oxygen radicals cause toxicity by way of varying mechanisms including lipid peroxidation, protein oxidation and DNA damage. In 1994, researchers O. Ben Yoseph and B.D. Ross at the Department of Radiology and Biological Chemistry at the University of Michigan, conducted a study to determine whether the use of polyethylene glycol, which competently produces reactive oxygen species, combined with glucose oxidase (GO) creates the cytotoxic environment needed to successfully treat solid tumors.

Two intra-tumoral injections were administered to lab rats and the results showed a significant delay in the growth of the tumors. This study suggests that oxidation therapy that combines the use of intra-tumoral ROS-generating enzymes for treating solid tumors is a promising area that needs additional research.

Study #2

In 2008, a study performed by K. Yoshizaki, T. Fujiki, et al. at Kyushu University in Japan investigated whether mild oxidative stress would trigger aging in human tumor cells, such as lung adenocarcinoma. The results showed that sub-lethal concentrations of hydrogen peroxide induced aging in cells and helped to make them weaker, but did not totally eliminate the tumors.

To gain a better understanding why this occurred, researchers investigated the outcome of the study. The results suggested that the cells treated with hydrogen peroxide were composed of heterogeneous cells; some were sensitive to hydrogen peroxide, while the others were resistant to it and reverted to their original tumorigenic forms. This research suggests that to properly treat cancerous tumors, the molecular mechanisms responsible for determining cellular fate should first be identified. Only then can researchers utilize the aging process of the tumor as one method for successfully inhibiting its growth.

As you can see there have been several successful studies on H_2O_2 therapy and its potential for cancer treatment. Some of these studies involved humans others involved animals, but the results hold much promise. While there is still a lot of on-going research, it is nice to know that there is an alternative to aggressive therapies like chemotherapy and radiation for individuals suffering from such debilitating and life-threatening conditions.

Differences between Food Grade Hydrogen Peroxide and Topical Hydrogen Peroxide

Many people assume that food grade hydrogen peroxide (also referred to as FGHP) and regular hydrogen peroxide (referred to as RHP, which is also the form most commonly found in homes across America) are the same. On the contrary, there are quite a few differences between these two forms of hydrogen peroxide.

A list of qualities and differences of FGHP and RHP is provided below.

Food Grade Hydrogen Peroxide (FGHP)

The FDA regulates the processing of food grade hydrogen peroxide (FGHP) and it undergoes a strict inspection process. If it does not pass inspection, it is no longer considered food grade hydrogen peroxide.

Food grade hydrogen peroxide comes in two different concentrations; 35 percent and 50 percent. This grade of H_2O_2 has no impurities, unlike the H_2O_2 purchased in the store.

FGHP is the type of hydrogen peroxide that can be used internally. However, **you must use extreme caution when handling and mixing it because it is extremely volatile.**

Food grade hydrogen peroxide is ideal for patients with otherwise compromised immune systems, such as people suffering from AIDS and various forms of cancer. This is because they need to be more concerned about ingesting contaminants and other substances they put into their bodies. FGHP has no contaminants. This lack of foreign contaminants makes it safer for people with compromised immune systems to use, since they are less likely to be sickened by it.

Due to its higher concentration, 35 percent food grade hydrogen peroxide can produce promising results when applied and used correctly. It can be administered internally via injections, or intravenously - directly into the blood stream. It can even be ingested when diluted properly.

Household Hydrogen Peroxide

Regular H2O2 – the kind that can purchased at the grocery store - is usually 3% hydrogen peroxide. It is used to treat cuts, scrapes and wounds due to its antiseptic properties, and works as a sanitizing agent.

This type of hydrogen peroxide is made from 50 percent Super D Peroxide, Diluted. This grade of hydrogen peroxide contains stabilizers such as acetanilide, phenol, terasodium phosphate and sodium stannate. It also contains some contaminants, which won't be harmful to otherwise healthy people. However, it should never be consumed!

Medical Application of Hydrogen Peroxide

Both regular grade hydrogen peroxide and food grade hydrogen peroxide are multipurpose. However, it is important to note that only Food Grade Hydrogen Peroxide should be ingested or used internally.

Common Uses for 3 Percent (Store Bought) Hydrogen Peroxide

Soaked with a Cotton Ball

When you scraped your knee or cut your finger, your mom may have soaked a cotton ball with hydrogen peroxide and placed it on your injury. This is because 3 percent grade hydrogen peroxide is great for killing bacteria, and prevents cuts and wounds from becoming infected.

As an All-Natural Foot Soak

Store bought hydrogen peroxide can also be diluted with water and used as an all-natural solution to soak your feet in. It alleviates painful corns and calluses by softening the dead, rough skin on the sides and bottom of the feet. It can also be used to treat minor cuts and abrasions.

Mixed with water

You can use a weak solution of hydrogen peroxide to boost the natural highlights and lowlights of your hair color.

As an All-Natural Cleansing Agent

The book "Hydrogen Peroxide: Medical Miracle," suggests soaking or dipping your toothbrushes in 3% hydrogen peroxide after each use to kill bacteria that accumulates on your toothbrush. You can treat yourself to a fresh toothbrush everyday by taking the time to do this between brushings.

As an Oral Mouth Rinse

According to the book "Hydrogen Peroxide: Medical Miracle," many people also use store bought hydrogen peroxide as an oral mouth rinse. H2O2 helps to kill bad breath germs just as effectively as or even better than mouthwash. Many people use it to treat halitosis, which is a health condition that causes offensive, odorous bad breath. Just take about two tablespoons of H2O2 into the mouth, swish it around and spit it out. Make sure you do not swallow it.

For More Severe Bad Breath

If you suffer from severe bad breath due to sinus problems, you can also utilize H2O2 to help reduce the smell of your breath. The book "Hydrogen Peroxide: Medical Miracle," suggests **diluting 3% store bought hydrogen peroxide** to half-strength using water. Once you do this, **place 5 to 10 drops in each nostril**. Make sure you **sniff the solution vigorously** to ensure it gets into the sinus cavities. Keep in mind that it will burn slightly as you inhale it! Do this treatment **twice a day**. If this helps cure your bad breath, you know it was sinus-related.

As a Homemade Toothpaste

HPS-online.com suggests mixing a few drops of hydrogen peroxide with a few teaspoons of water, a dash of salt and a dash of baking soda to make your own toothpaste. This toothpaste will help to whiten teeth and prevent bad breath.

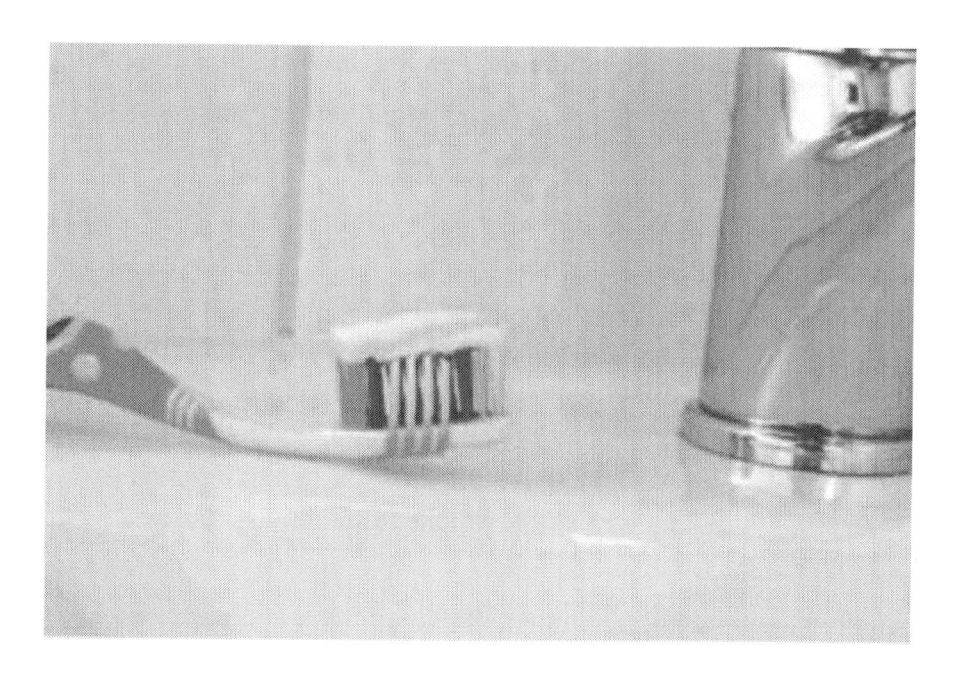

Common Uses for 30 Percent Grade (Food Grade) Hydrogen Peroxide

To Treat Influenza and Pneumonia

A **food grade hydrogen peroxide** solution of 0.03 percent is often administered intravenously. It is allowed to infuse slowly into a patient's vein for a period of one to three hours.

Treatments may be given once a week for more acute illnesses, but they can also be given daily for influenza or pneumonia. Intravenous hydrogen peroxide treatments can range from as little as one treatment to as many as 20 doses. Keep in mind, though, that the range of treatment depends on the severity of the illness and overall health of the patient.

To Loosen Mucus Deep within the Lungs

Once the hydrogen peroxide is injected into the diseased area, such as the lungs, the substance begins to bubble and loosen the mucus, detaching it from the lining of the lungs. The patient then coughs up the mucus and other debris from within the lungs. Only a highly trained professional or doctor should administer hydrogen peroxide intravenously, since it is highly toxic if not diluted to the proper concentration or administered properly.

To Treat Rheumatoid and Osteoarthritis

Food grade hydrogen peroxide can also be administered by way of injections. Usually this solution consists of 0.03 percent hydrogen peroxide, which is injected directly into the inflamed joint. Hydrogen peroxide therapy injections are often used to treat both rheumatoid and osteoarthritis.

To Treat Stiff Joints, Fungal Infections and Skin Conditions

Properly diluted food grade hydrogen peroxide can also be used topically to treat stiff joints, in addition to fungal infections and skin conditions such as psoriasis.

To Help Improve Oxygen Circulation in the Body

An easy way to absorb hydrogen peroxide through the skin is by taking a bath in diluted 30 percent food grade hydrogen peroxide. This will help to open up the pores so oxygen can circulate more freely throughout the skin.

To Open Up Airways in the Lungs and Remove Toxins from the Skin

Many people ingest H2O2, **but only after it has been diluted**. You can dilute 30% FGHP to 3% by mixing it with water. It will then be safe to drink. When the hydrogen peroxide is ingested, it helps to open up the lungs and even has benefits for the skin.

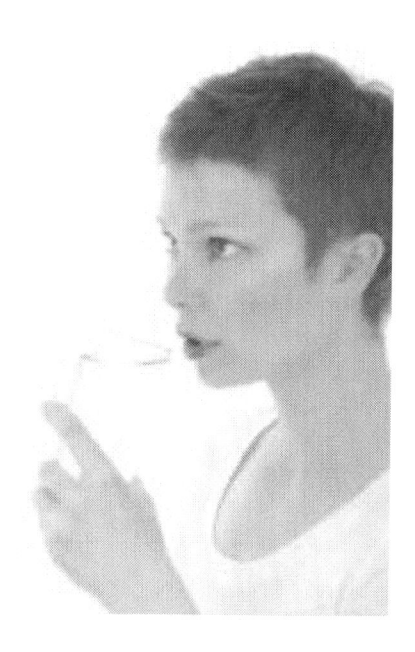

To Improve Lung Functioning

Many people utilize a regular nasal spray pump to administer H_2O_2 treatments. You can purchase one at a medical supply store or you may already have one in your house. If you already have one, you'll need to empty out the contents and sterilize the bottle before you add the solution to it. You can wash it out with antibacterial soap and water and allow it to air dry before you pour the food grade H_2O_2 solution in it.

As an Overnight Breathing Treatment

According to the book, "Hydrogen Peroxide for Health," you can use diluted food grade hydrogen peroxide as a breathing treatment by placing 1 oz. of food grade hydrogen peroxide along with a gallon of water inside a humidifier or vaporizer and allowing it to run the entire night.

This treatment helps improve lung functioning and breathing, so you'll feel refreshed and rejuvenated. Many people also claim that it helps put an end to their snoring.

To Treat Vaginal Infections

Food grade H2O2 has also been used to help treat a variety of vaginal infections. It helps to kill the fungi and bacteria that cause these infections while maintaining proper pH balance of good bacteria.

Different Grades of Hydrogen Peroxide and Their Uses

Once you decide to try one of the many types of hydrogen peroxide treatment that we've discussed, you must choose which grade of hydrogen peroxide will work best for what your needs. It is extremely important to remember that only Food Grade Hydrogen Peroxide should be ingested or administered internally.

Below is a list of different grades of hydrogen peroxide and their uses.

- **3 Percent Pharmaceutical Grade-** The most common form of hydrogen peroxide, which is carried at most drugstores. No prescription is needed. It can be used externally to treat cuts, scrapes, and wounds, but should never be used internally because it contains many different stabilizers that can be toxic.

- **6 Percent Beautician Grade-** Many hairstylists and beauticians use hydrogen peroxide of this grade as a solution to lighten hair. It should never be ingested, especially since it can potentially contain bleach and stabilizers.

- **30 Percent Reagent Grade-** This grade of hydrogen peroxide is used in a variety of scientific experiments; however, it also contains stabilizers and is therefore not designed to be used internally.

- **30 to 32 Percent Electronic Grade-** This grade of H2O2 is utilized to clean electronics and should not be used internally.

- **35 Percent Technical Grade-** While hydrogen peroxide of this grade is comparable to Reagent grade, it is more heavily concentrated. It also contains phosphorus, which helps to neutralize chemicals like chlorine within the water that is added to it. Do not ingest or use this grade internally.

- **35 Percent Food Grade-** This is the only grade suggested for internal administration and ingestion. Since this grade has antiseptic properties, it is used to spray the foil lining of boxed juice products and in the production of dairy products.

Safe Administration of Hydrogen Peroxide Therapy

"Do not try this without consulting with your doctor first!!!!

You should always use chlorine-free, distilled water when you decide to administering H2O2 treatment. Distilled water is free from impurities; an essential requirement for the treatment to work the way it was intended.

To make the hydrogen peroxide solution, pour 1 ounce of 35 percent food grade H2O2 into a jar that measures 1 pint. Add 11 ounces of distilled water to the H2O2. This will make 12 ounces of 3% H2O2.

Inhalation Method

Use the food grade hydrogen peroxide solution that is diluted with water so that it is 3% concentrated. Fill the spray bottle pump with the solution and insert it into your mouth. Pump the solution into your mouth about 5 to 10 times and inhale deeply at the same time you do this. Repeat this treatment twice a day, two times in the morning and two times in the late afternoon.

If you recently have been ill, consider administering the treatment every four to six hours.

Transdermal Application

You can also hydrogen peroxide by bathing in it. This can be accomplished by adding 1 to 8 pints of 3% solution to a bathtub filled with lukewarm water.

Vaporizer Method

Your breathing can benefit if you add food grade H2O2 to a humidifier or vaporizer. Many people add 15 ounces of 3 percent food grade hydrogen peroxide to 1 gallon of water. This method has been touted for its benefits on lung function, and some users claim that it has even put an end to their snoring.

Topical Application

Podiatry patients are often given a foot soak that consists of a tub of warm water and one pint of 35 percent **food grade hydrogen peroxide**. They are instructed to soak their feet in this solution for approximately 20 minutes. This application helps to get rid of athlete's foot fungi and bacteria that fester between the toes.

Douche

If you experience a bacterial infection down under, you can add three tablespoons of the 3 percent H2O2 solution to a quart of distilled water. This solution will help to kill the bacteria that are responsible for vaginal infections.

Proper Dilution for Food Grade Hydrogen Therapy

If you plan to ingest hydrogen peroxide, the only form you should consider using is 35 percent food-grade formula. However, you should never use it without diluting it first. Even food grade hydrogen peroxide of 10 percent, if ingested, can cause serious brain damage. It is also extremely volatile, so you should be extremely careful when handling or mixing it.

If 35% H2O2 makes contact with your skin it will cause a chemical burn, so you'll want to rinse the area thoroughly with water. You also want to follow the guidelines precisely when you decide to mix and administer it. Many people find it easier to administer diluted hydrogen peroxide by using an eyedropper and dipping it inside of a glass container.

Duration of H2O2 Therapy

Always work with a trained medical professional to create a treatment plan that is suitable for you!!!!

The length of time that a person stays on oxygen therapy is dependent on their overall health and what conditions they are treating. For acute diseases and illnesses, the treatment and the dosage should be higher and more frequent. You should maintain the maximum dosage for at least one week if your condition is mild. For more severe illnesses, stay on the maximum dosage for up to 21 days.

According to HPS-online.com, when using higher dosages to treat more severe illnesses, you'll want to use more water to dilute the H2O2, and always make sure to stay at 25 drops, administered 3 times a day for a minimum of 1 to 3 weeks. Then gradually decrease the dosage to 25 drops, administered 2 times a day, until you no longer experience any symptoms of the illness or health problem you are treating. This can take anywhere from 1 to 6 months, so hang in there!

When you no longer have any symptoms of the illness or health condition you are treating, you can begin tapering off treatment. HPS-online.com suggests following the schedule below:

25 drops, one time every other day, 4 times
25 drops, once every third day for 14 days
25 drops once every fourth day for 21 days

An ideal maintenance schedule to follow would be between 5 to 15 drops a week, dependent upon how many processed foods and cooked foods you consume on a daily basis.

If for any reason you experience an upset stomach during any level of administration, you have two choices: you can decide to stay on that current level of treatment until you feel that it is necessary to stop, or you can decrease your dosage by going back one level.

Those patients suffering from candida may need to start treatment at 1 drop administered 3 times daily.

Storage and Safety Tips

Many unfortunate and dangerous accidents can occur if proper safety precautions are not followed when mixing, administering and storing FG hydrogen peroxide. For this particular reason, it is essential that you read and follow these safety and storage tips **exactly as they are given.**

Make sure to read these instructions thoroughly before mixing and administering FGH2O2 treatment, and refer to them whenever you need clarification.

1. Keep H2O2 concentrate out of the reach of children.
2. Never place concentrate inside of unlabeled or improperly labeled jars or containers.
3. If pure H2O2 makes contact with the skin, flush the area immediately with water.
4. If undiluted H2O2 is accidentally ingested, drink numerous glasses of water to help dilute it. Stay in an upright position and contact your medical provider immediately. It can be fatal if swallowed at full strength.
5. To dispose of hydrogen peroxide properly, please refer to the local, state, and federal regulations.
6. Flush the area where hydrogen peroxide was spilled with water. Do not place any spilled material back into the original container. Instead, report spills according to regulations put forth by local, state, and federal agencies.
7. Large quantities of hydrogen peroxide should be stored in an area or environment that is cool and dry.
8. Be careful not to allow FG H2O2 to come into contact with organic materials, as this can cause spontaneous combustion.
9. Small quantities of 35 percent FGHP should be wrapped with black plastic wrap, labeled, and stored in the freezer.
10. 35 percent FGHP won't freeze unless the temperature falls to 33 degrees below zero.
11. Lower concentrations of FG H2O2 such as 3 or 6 percent will freeze; therefore, storing these concentrations in the freezer is not recommended.
12. Label containers and store them in a cool dry place, where children

cannot gain access to them.

First Aid and Emergency Procedures

EYES:

Flush with water instantly for a length of 15 minutes or more and make sure to take turns lifting and cleansing the upper and lower eyelids while rinsing. Go to the nearest hospital for examination and correct treatment.

SKIN:

Wash the infected area thoroughly with soap and water. Seek medical attention if irritation or pain exists.

INGESTION:

Rinse mouth thoroughly with water. Dilute the swallowed solution by drinking 1 to 2 glasses of water. Never induce vomiting.

Never attempt to give a person any liquids if they are unconscious. Seek medical attention immediately.

INHALATION:

Move to an area outside, where there is plenty of fresh air. If breathing becomes labored or discomfort continues, contact a medical professional immediately.

NOTICE TO MEDICAL DOCTOR:

Undiluted H_2O_2 that is ingested is a powerful oxidant. If these concentrations accidentally make contact with the eyes, they can damage the cornea, especially when it is not washed immediately after exposure. It is highly advised that a careful ophthalmologic exam is conducted and possible local corticosteroid therapy be administered.

It is suggested that evacuating the stomach by way of gastric lavage or emesis induction be avoided, since systemic effects and corrosive effects on the gastrointestinal tract can occur. One possible treatment for ingested undiluted H_2O_2 is the insertion of an orogastric or nasogastric tube, which might be required to reduce severe distension caused by gas formation.

If accidental contact of food grade H_2O_2 is made at full strength, you should follow the first aid procedures given by this booklet or guidelines provided by your Federal, State and local agencies.

Conclusion

Hydrogen peroxide plays a pivotal role in the human body. Not only does hydrogen peroxide occur naturally within the body, but different grades are scientifically engineered, and each one serves its own purpose.

While the only form of hydrogen peroxide that should be consumed is food grade hydrogen peroxide, it should never be consumed at full strength. It should always be properly diluted, first. Other forms of hydrogen peroxide exist, but most of these concentrations are made specifically for industrial use and should never be ingested or consumed. The amount of hydrogen peroxide that occurs within the human body is essential for the proper functioning of all cells, and it has also been used in various research studies to help medical professionals find alternative ways to treat minor and acute diseases and illnesses.

Hydrogen peroxide helps doctors and researchers provide people with a natural treatment alternative for various heart conditions by helping to clear the arteries, which allows oxygen and blood to flow more freely, in turn improving circulation and overall health of people suffering from these illnesses and diseases.

H2O2 also helps to fight fungal, bacterial and viral infections because it not only has antiseptic properties; it also increases the amount of oxygen within the blood. Many people believe that viruses and dysfunctional cells such as those found in cancer cannot survive or thrive in an oxygen-abundant environment.

Hydrogen peroxide therapy has been used to help treat different types of arthritis and other forms of inflammation. H2O2 prevents inflammation from occurring by controlling the problem that is responsible for causing inflammation.

H2O2 therapy has also been shown to be an effective treatment for various lung diseases such as emphysema, COPD, and bronchitis. It helps to clear air passages by breaking up the mucous deep within the lungs, which can become infected. The patient is then able to cough up the debris and expel it from the body, thus decreasing the risk of further infections. Once this is done, breathing is improved and the person no longer experiences problems breathing.

Some people even claim to no longer have a problem with snoring once they administer H2O2 therapy, as a result of cleared nasal passages and improved breathing.

Since FG H2O2 in pure form is highly volatile, it should be handled with care and proper handling, mixing and storing instructions should be followed exactly.

This fact cannot be emphasized enough: **proper dilution of H2O2 is required in order for the treatment to work the way it was intended.**

Even healthy people may experience side effects of FG H2O2 treatment. This treatment works by helping the body expel toxins such as viruses, diseases and illnesses, which might affect some more than others. Stop the treatment immediately and see a doctor if you react strongly to H2O2.

If the person continues to experience these uncomfortable symptoms, they can choose to either stay on the treatment or reduce the dosage and the amount of times they take it each day.

H2O2 therapy should be taken on an empty stomach **or** three hours after you have eaten. It should also be taken in the morning and/or mid-afternoon. When the body experiences an increase in oxygen and improved circulation, people may find that they have more energy which is beneficial when they first wake up in the morning, but can interfere with their ability to fall asleep and stay asleep.

Online Sources

http://www.atsdr.cdc.gov/tfacts174.pdf

http://curezone.com/forums/fm.asp?i=1470131#I

http://www.coolscience.org/CoolScience/KidScientists/h2o2.htm

http://www.chemsystems.com/about/cs/news/items/PERP%200708_3_Hydrogen%20Peroxide.cfm

http://cira.ornl.gov/documents/HydrogenPeroxide.pdf

http://www.biology-online.org/dictionary/Photolysis

http://www.biology-online.org/dictionary/Endogenous

http://www.rcsb.org/pdb/101/motm.do?momID=57

http://educate-yourself.org/cancer/benefitsofhydrogenperozide17jul03.shtml

http://www.hps-online.com/hoxy.htm

http://www.the-natural-path.com/hydrogen-peroxide-therapy.html

http://www.foodgrade-hydrogenperoxide.com/id32.html

http://www.arthritistrust.org/Articles/Hydrogen%20Peroxide%20Therapy.pdf

http://www.drhui.com/?page_id=41

http://www.lenntech.com/processes/disinfection/chemical/disinfectants-hydrogen-peroxide.htm

http://www.ncbi.nlm.nih.gov/pubmed/11544023

http://www.medterms.com/script/main/art.asp?articlekey=11287

http://www.ncbi.nlm.nih.gov/pubmed/21148404

http://www.foodgrade-hydrogenperoxide.com/sitebuildercontent/sitebuilderfiles/TheTruthAboutFGHP.pdf

http://www.ehow.com/about_6523764_glucose-oxidase_.html

http://www.vanderbilt.edu/AnS/psychology/health_psychology/oxygen.htm

http://www.integrativemed.com/resources/HydrogenPeroxide.pdf

http://www.maebrussell.com/Health/Oxygen%20Therapies.html

http://www.scribd.com/doc/49600371/7/The-Farr-Experiments

http://www.nlm.nih.gov/medlineplus/ency/article/003333.htm

http://www.umm.edu/ency/article/003333.htm

http://medical-dictionary.thefreedictionary.com/gamma+globulin

http://www.emedicinehealth.com/candidiasis_yeast_infection/article_em.htm

http://www.ncbi.nlm.nih.gov/pubmedhealth/PMH0004449/

http://www.foodgrade-hydrogenperoxide.com/id31.html

http://www.earthclinic.com/Remedies/hydrogen_peroxide_inhalation.html

http://www.h2o2-4u.com/grades.html

http://educate-yourself.org/fc/

http://uuhsc.utah.edu/poison/healthpros/utox/toxtoday/Vol10_Iss1.pdf

http://www.scribd.com/doc/11632119/Hydrogen-Peroxide-For-Health

http://medical-dictionary.thefreedictionary.com/Ozone+Therapy

http://www.hps-online.com/hoxy.htm

http://msds.fmc.com/msds/100000010225-MSDS_US-E.pdf

http://www.drceaser.com/therapies/intravenous-hydrogen-peroxide-therapy

http://educate-yourself.org/cn/hydrogenperoxidecancertherapybookexcerpt.shtml

Book Sources

Schlager, N. & Weisblatt, J. (2006). Chemical Compounds. Volume 2: Ethyl Alcohol-Polysiloxane. Montney, C.B. (Ed.), (pp. 363-366). Thomson Gale.

Journal Sources

Del Rio, M.J. (2004). The Hydrogen Peroxide and its Importance in Alzheimer's and Parkinson's Disease. Current Medicinal Chemistry-Central Nervous System Agents, 4 (4), 279-285.

Munakata, T., Semba,U. et al. (1985). Induction of Interferon-gamma Production by Human Natural Killer Cells Stimulated by Hydrogen Peroxide, *Journal of Immunology*, 134(4), 2449-2455.

Elevated levels of urinary hydrogen peroxide, advanced oxidative protein product (AOPP) and malondialdehyde in humans infected with intestinal parasites, (2009). *Parasitology*, 136 (3), 359-363.

Lopes, F., Coelho, F., et al. (2011). Resolution of Europhilic inflammation by H2O2 in antigen-induced arthritis. *Arthritis & Rheumatism*, 63, (9), 2651-2660.

Vassalle, C., Landi, P., et al. (2007). Oxidative stress evaluated using an automated method for hydro peroxide estimation in patients with coronary artery disease. *Clinical Chemistry & Laboratory Medicine*, 45 (3), 367-371.

Capizzi, R., Landi, F., et al. (2004). Skin tolerability and efficacy of combination therapy with hydrogen peroxide stabilized cream and adapalene gel in comparison with benzoyl peroxide cream and adapalene gel in common acne. A randomized, investigator-masked, controlled trial. *British Journal of Dermatology*, 151 (2), 481-484.

Ben-Yoseph, O., & Ross, B.D., (1994). Oxidation therapy: the use of a reactive oxygen species-generating enzyme system for tumour treatment. Departments of Radiology and Biological Chemistry, University of Michigan, Krese III Research Building, Room R3315, Ann Arbor, Michigan

Yoshizaki, K., Fujiki, T., et al. (2008). Pro-Senescent Effect of Hydrogen Peroxide on Cancer Cells and Its Possible Application to Tumour Suppression. Department of Genetic Resources Technology, faculty of Agriculture, Kyushu University, Japan.

Printed in Great Britain
by Amazon.co.uk, Ltd.,
Marston Gate.